I0440109

ENLIGHTENING GUIDE TO PCOS

What is Polycystic Ovarian Syndrome?

Dr. Linda J Howland
PhD Biomed. Sci.

Amazon Edition
First Edition eBook – 2014

Acknowledgements

The *Health Hunter* series of books are dedicated to the gorgeous women of the world, whose strength, beauty, confidence and intelligence should be celebrated every day. This book is dedicated to my two beautiful children, who have taught me more about love than I ever knew was possible. Who continue to make me laugh and learn, fall down and get up again, to appreciate the small things in life and the importance of family in what ever form it takes. Love you to bits.

A huge heart felt thanks to my friends and family for their support and assistance in helping to champion my passion and purpose, encouraging me to focus it into creating this e-book series. Most of all, I must express much gratitude and love to my husband Jay. Whose dedication, focus and drive is an inspiration to me everyday, and whose love and support means the world to me.

With much gratitude and best wishes for great health and happiness for all,

Dr. Linda Howland.

Forward: A note from the Author

After many years of struggling with my own health and finding more questions than answers as I walked out from the multitude of health visits, I decided it was time to use my skills and passion as a medical researcher to empower myself and others to live happy and healthy lives as PCOS women. Always a "searcher" and fuelled by my own frustration, I was determined not to give up. I had also realised that it was up to me to take responsibility for my own health because – let's face it – no one cares more about the health of *your body* than *you*! I began to hunt and gather any credible sources of information about PCOS. The results are simplified and jam packed into this neat three part series of e-books, instantly ready for you to download and devour the information in your own time. The information is presented in a simplified way and often includes examples, but I also wanted to provide detailed knowledge that can empower you to lead a healthy and happy life with PCOS.

After speaking with numerous friends, family and acquaintances with PCOS, I found there was a huge gap in the information being provided to newly diagnosed women with PCOS. It appeared there was a lack of information or that it was delivered in a complex way. As a medical researcher, I knew that exciting new information was being discovered by clinical researchers and not reaching the women who would find it most beneficial. I felt the strong obligation to share this news with my fellow PCOS ladies. The outcome is to empower you to make positive health choices through knowledge and self-management in concert with the advice of your chosen health professionals and ultimately allow you to be in control of your health and happiness. You could think of this as you becoming the driver (rather than the passenger) of your body and of your health professionals as your expert race support team.

Knowledge is power, and when it comes to understanding your body, it allows you and your team of chosen health professionals to construct a personalised health plan that aims to restore vitality and total wellbeing. Don't be afraid of your health care professionals. They are there to help you but it's just as important to step up and help yourself! Don't be afraid to ask questions, push for answers or request tests if you believe they are necessary or informative. Always seek a second or third opinion if you feel you are not receiving the best level of care or don't feel comfortable to explore your health concerns fully with your current health professional. Importantly, don't let a professional dismiss your concerns with archaic misinformation, such as "you're too slim to have PCOS" or "don't worry about it until you want to have kids some day down the track". As revealed in this e-book series, there is far more to PCOS than just having "lumpy ovaries" and early diagnosis may give you the head start you need to keep your health on track, regain balance and prevent serious health problems later in life.

The *Health Hunter* series of health information e-books was created to help equip individuals with the power of knowledge, enabling them to make pivotal decisions about their health and to make sense of the health resources readily available to them. This information in turn can be shared with friends and families to help them make better choices too. At the end of the day, it's your body, your health, your life, and your future that's at stake.

Knowledge empowers you to understand your condition, ask the right questions, request the right tests from your chosen health professionals and understand the results. It's so important to become aware and take personal responsibility.

This means using what you learn to then take action and make the changes required to turn your life around, allowing you to live life to the fullest and become the positive, healthy, happy and energetic person you deserve to be.

Sincerely and with much gratitude and goodwill,
Dr. Linda Howland

Table of Contents

Acknowledgements	2
Forward: A note from the Author	3
Table of Contents	6
Disclaimer	7
Copyright	8
PCOS – Understanding the condition	**9**
What is Polycystic Ovarian Syndrome?	*10*
What are the symptoms or complications of PCOS?	*16*
Disrupted hormones and the effects on the female body	*19*
Diagnosis/Testing for PCOS	**21**
PCO versus PCOS	*21*
What tests are used to confirm you have PCOS?	*22*
Different types of PCOS	*29*
Why me? What causes PCOS?	**32**
Genetic factors that could be causing PCOS	*34*
Environmental factors that could be causing PCOS	*46*
Living to your full potential with PCOS	**54**
Concluding remarks	**55**
Other e-books in the Health Hunter Books series	*56*
Join the conversation	*57*
References	**58**

Disclaimer

The author does not dispense medical advice or prescribe the use of any method or techniques for the treatment of a physical, emotional or medical problem. The advice provided in this article is for informational purposes only. This document is designed to provide information to assist decision-making. It is based on the best available evidence and clinical research at the time of development of this publication. It is not meant to augment nor replace consultation with a licensed health care provider.

Consultation with a health care provider or other primary care provider is highly recommended for anyone suffering from a health problem. Any advice given in this publication is to be followed subject to the clinician's judgment and patient's preference in each individual case.

Due to the ever-changing nature of the Internet, web addresses or links contained in this book may have changed since publication and, as such, may not be valid. Any imagery of people used within this book was purchased and are of models. As such, all images are used for illustrative purposes only and any person depicted in the content, if any, is a model.

Copyright

PCOS – Understanding the condition

Congratulations! Reading this e-book is your first step to hunting down the latest information about polycystic ovarian syndrome (PCOS). Using this resource in conjunction with gathering a team of knowledgeable health professionals will help you set up your game plan and then kick it into action so you can get on living a happy and health life with PCOS.

The first book in this three-part e-book series about PCOS will help you to gain an understanding of PCOS in terms of what is going on in your body. It will explain what symptoms and problems PCOS may be causing, how these are used to diagnose the condition and other tests that can be done by medical practitioners to help you create a clear and personal diagnosis of your PCOS condition. PCOS can vary from person to person and therefore changes the way you need to treat or manage the condition. I've also included some recent information from experts in the field on how it came to be that you are living with this condition and how these genetic or environmental factors may also be affecting your health in other ways that are just as crucial to your health.

The second and third e-books in this series will reveal the current and new strategies for managing PCOS including both traditional and alternative options, and also how this may influence your fertility and health as you age. Living life as a woman who is Powerfully Capable of Obtaining Success (my preferred use of the acronym PCOS) means taking personal responsibility for managing your health and wellbeing, so congratulations again for actively seeking knowledge to empower your choices.

What is Polycystic Ovarian Syndrome?

Polycystic Ovary (Ovarian) Syndrome (PCOS) is a very common disorder that affects the reproductive (sex) organs of women. Basically, it is a condition that disrupts your sex hormones and the systems they control.

How common is PCOS?

PCOS is a very common condition for women. It affects 12-21% of women who are of reproductive age in Australia [1]. That's at least one in every ten women. Recent studies suggest it is likely to be one in every five women of reproductive age, making it more than half a million Australian women with PCOS.

It was first described by doctors in the 1930s and has also been referred to as "Stein Leventhal Syndrome" (after the two American guys who first described it in 1935) "Hyperandrogen Anovulation Syndrome" or "Polycystic Ovarian Disorder (PCOD)". Although common in women, it often goes undetected or undiagnosed.

In Australia it is estimated that 70% of women with PCOS may have the condition but don't know it [2]. For example, in a room full of 30 women, one of them is likely to have been diagnosed with PCOS, but another two are completely unaware that they also have the condition. Without proper management, these two women may potentially be sitting on a biological time bomb or suffering with the side effects of PCOS without realising there are options available to them to manage the condition and improve their health and happiness.

What's the problem?

Although we now have a better understanding of what changes are present in the body of a woman with PCOS, what exactly causes PCOS (its pathophysiology) still remains a mystery. Experts currently believe that both your genetics and/or environmental factors play a role [3,4] and that these changes are closely linked with the insulin pathway (more commonly associated with diabetes).

Regardless of the cause, what is known for sure is that PCOS is the result of long-term (chronic) disruptions to the endocrine system causing an imbalance of sex hormones.

The endocrine system is a network of glands that secrete chemicals into the body. These chemicals act as messengers to control and coordinate all the parts of the body. You could think of this system as the "Post Office" of your body. Think of the individual glands as the post offices, and the chemical messengers as the letters being sent all around the body to different organs. Organs (like your heart, skin etc.) are made up of lots of individual cells, similar to a household with lots of individual people living in one house. Just like receiving a letter that tells you to do something, like pay a bill, when a cell comes in contact with a chemical messenger it tells it what to do. For example grow, shrink, die, secrete something, and many other interesting functions that coordinate together to produce all the amazing functions of the beautiful body you live in. Disruptions to this system, as occurs in PCOS, can cause chaos and imbalances in your body.

What are hormones and how do they work?

Hormones are a special type of chemical messenger produced by the endocrine system. They are responsible for many important functions in the body including growth, breathing, digestion, stress, sleep and even your mood. Hormones produce their effects by docking with matching receptors on or inside a cell (like putting a key into a lock of a door). What is special about hormones is that they need to be released in the correct amount (usually minute quantities) and pattern in order to produce the right responses in the body. For example, hormones control your monthly reproductive cycle (your period).

For women with PCOS, the endocrine system doesn't produce or respond to hormones correctly. In particular, there is an imbalance in the amounts or responses to sex hormones (estrogen, progesterone and testosterone). So you could say the post office is experiencing a delivery failure because it keeps sending the same mail, the mailbox can't be found, or the messages keep getting received as junk and not taken seriously.

Regardless of whether or not the exact fault is identified, the outcome is the same. A communication break down that disrupts normal function and balance in the body.

What are sex hormones and what do they do?

Sex hormones are powerful chemical messengers produced by the sex organs. The ovaries are the sex organs in women, and the testes are the sex organs in men. Both men and women also release sex hormones from their adrenal glands. The balance of sex hormones estrogen and testosterone regulate the functions of the reproductive system and are responsible for making the characteristic and biological differences between men and women. In simple terms, women have higher levels of estrogen and men have higher levels of testosterone.

The brain releases control hormones that travel through the blood to reach the sex organs (ovaries, testes) where they stimulate the production and release of sex hormones. Sex hormones affect many different functions in the body including growth, your appearance and reproduction. They can also influence other systems of the body like the immune system. When they are disrupted in women with PCOS, they cause a variety of annoying and disruptive symptoms all over the body, including, but not exclusively, the development of polycystic ovaries (PCO).

Where are the ovaries and what do they do?

Ovaries are the sex organs for women and they produce the sex hormones as well as release mature ovum (eggs) for conception. For women, the reproductive tract consists of a series of tubes that lead from the vaginal entrance up to the two ovaries. From the vaginal entrance, the tract leads up past the narrow canal of the cervix, and into the uterus. The uterus is lined with a thick layer of cells called the endometrium, which is shed each month during your period if pregnancy doesn't occur. Off each side of the uterus are two fallopian tubes (like arms), which stretch out with finger like projections to the ovaries.

Inside the ovaries the ovum (eggs) are matured roughly once a month, alternating from side to side, and a single egg (in most cases) is released into the tract where it has the opportunity to meet up with sperm if unprotected sex has occurred recently. If no sperm is present, the egg will not be fertilised and this signals for your period to occur shortly after.

As mentioned before, the ovaries also produce and release the sex hormones in response to chemical messages sent from the brain. A normal ovary is about the size and shape of an almond (3 to 5 cm in length) but becomes smaller following menopause. They are dark grey/black in colour with small bumps on the surface. A polycystic ovary (PCO) is often larger and has numerous large bumps that look like cysts covering the surface.

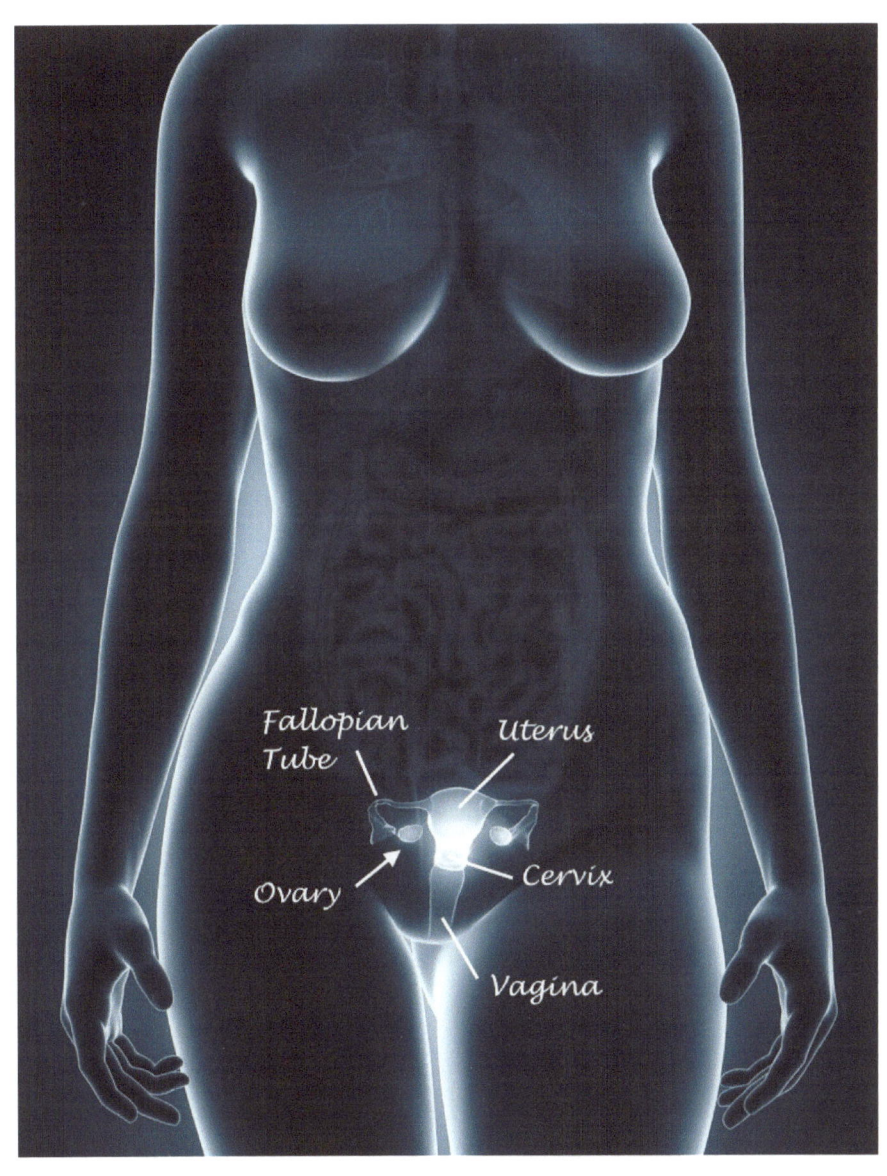

The Female Reproductive Tract
Copyright adapted from Shutterstock.com/154771646

What are the symptoms or complications of PCOS?

The way PCOS presents in the body will vary from one person to another (referred to as a heterogeneous disease). The symptoms may include changes in the following:

Elevated levels of sex hormones (estrogen and testosterone) in your body, particularly higher levels of androgens (male-related sex hormones) like testosterone. These hormones can be fproduced in higher levels by the body. Or are just not bound up the way they should be to receptors on cells or hormone binding proteins present in the body, and so they remain "free" and active in the blood. This can increase their effects. This higher level of sex hormones can then cause changes to your appearance and menstrual cycles (as explained further below).

Masculisation occurs in women when excess androgen (male sex hormones) is present. The clinical evidence includes acne, alopecia in addition to hirsutism. This is different to virilisation, which occurs in more severe hyperandrogenism and causes temporal balding, deepening of the voice, increased muscle bulk, and clitoromegaly. This is very uncommon for women with PCOS. These are more likely to be the clinical signs of Hyperthecosis, a condition where the ovaries contain extra theca cells which produce androgens and more often occurs in post-menopausal women [6].

Changes to your menstrual cycle (commonly called your "period") can occur which may include more or less frequent times when an egg is released correctly from your ovaries (ovulation) and then how often your period occurs (when the egg is not fertilised and no pregnancy occurs). Periods are often irregular, infrequent or heavy for women with PCOS. Menstrual irregularity is described in more detail in the diagnosis and testing chapter.

The presence of polycystic ovaries (PCO) - A woman has two ovaries, one on each side of her uterus. When the eggs within the ovaries don't mature or get released incorrectly during ovulation, they form small follicles that look like (but aren't) cysts or fluid-filled sacs on the surface of the ovaries. These follicles can be seen in the ovaries using ultrasound examination and this is where the name polycystic ovaries come from. Unlike real ovarian cysts, immature follicles will not directly produce any harmful health problems and are thought to be more the result of mixed up hormonal signaling rather than the cause of PCOS and its related symptoms.

Fertility issues (subfertility) may be a problem arising from release of poor quality eggs or infrequent release of a mature egg from the ovaries each month and this will make it more challenging for a woman to become pregnant (but not impossible in most cases).

Changes in your appearance may occur, including the growth of excessive facial or body hair (hirsutism; 60%), usually in areas of male hair growth such as on the chin, cheeks, nipples, chest and back. This is the most common clinical sign that you have unusually high levels of male sex hormones in your body (hyperandrogenism) [5].

Another sign may be the presence of mild to severe acne on the face and body. Alopecia can also occur, which causes male-pattern baldness on the head. Enhanced sensitivity to testosterone by the cells in the body that normally respond to testosterone signals can also be the cause of these PCOS-induced changes to your appearance, so you may experience these symptoms but show normal testosterone levels in testing.

Increased insulin (sugar regulator) and weight problems are common in women with PCOS. Insulin is a hormone produced by your pancreas to help you convert sugar (glucose) and starches obtained from food (carbohydrates) into energy. Cells of the body, particularly the brain and the nervous system, use this glucose-derived energy to function. The liver, fat and muscle cells can take up the glucose and store it for release later. The hormone glucagon stimulates the release of this glucose from the cells in times when there is none available in the blood (when you have not eaten for a while). Thus, insulin and glucagon help keep the blood glucose levels balanced.

Women with PCOS often have high levels of insulin in their blood (hyper-insulinemia), which stimulate the ovaries to produce more testosterone, causing adverse changes to your appearance and menstrual cycle (explained in more detail further below). Chronic high levels of insulin can lead to insulin resistance (also referred to as metabolic syndrome) and type-2 diabetes. There is a greater chance of becoming overweight, particularly weight stored around the belly. This can happen when high insulin levels, combined with excessive food intake relative to the amount of exercise you are doing (energy in: energy out ratio), may mean that your cells receive more glucose than they need and so they convert it and store it as fat. Hence, it's easier to gain weight (fat) and harder to lose it (get the fat out of the cells).

Disrupted hormones and the effects on the female body

The large majority of women with PCOS will have more testosterone in their body than is needed. This is known as hyperandrogenism. One way this can happen is that the brain makes too much of a hormone called GnRH (Gonadotropin-Releasing Hormone). This hormone then makes another part of the brain release a different hormone called Luteinizing Hormone (LH). When LH reaches the ovaries (via the blood), it causes the theca cells inside the ovaries to produce testosterone.

Normally, if there were too much testosterone made by the ovaries, another hormone called FSH (follicle stimulating hormone) would tell the ovaries to break down the testosterone and make it into other types of sex hormones. However, in women with PCOS, the level of FSH is often too low. This leads to a build up of testosterone in the body.

Some PCOS women can also experience over activity of the enzymes responsible for producing testosterone in the ovarian cells, which provides another contributor to higher testosterone levels. In some cases, the adrenal glands may also be producing excess testosterone in addition to the activities of the ovaries.

No matter what the source of excess testosterone, the effects on the body remain the same. Testosterone in higher than normal levels creates an imbalance that causes changes in a woman's appearance, such as hirsutism (excessive hair growth), severe acne (on face and body), and alopecia (male pattern baldness).

The excess androgens can also be aromatised outside of the ovaries and be converted to estradiol and estrone, which can continue to stimulate the endometrium on the inside of the uterus to thicken. High levels of estradiol and progesterone would normally send a "feedback" message to the brain and signal for it to stop releasing GnRH, but the high levels of testosterone block the message getting there and results in excessive androgen production (a negative cycle).

There is also often a deficiency in progesterone that can contribute to this problem. Low progesterone can cause issues like trouble conceiving (frequent miscarriage), endometriosis, migraines, PMS, insulin resistance and weight gain [7].

Thus, treatment for PCOS often focuses on reducing the testosterone in the body to relieve the obvious physical symptoms (hair growth/loss, acne, etc.). However, if you want to manage both the adverse physical symptoms and metabolic problems related to PCOS or do all that and fall pregnant, it may be more beneficial to pursue other treatments that focus on restoring the balance to the ovulatory cycle whilst reducing the free testosterone levels.

Diagnosis/Testing for PCOS

Diagnosis is required to confirm that a woman has PCOS and not just PCO or other conditions that can be present and produce similar symptoms. The Rotterdam criteria are used to confirm if a woman has PCOS. Diagnosis can be difficult and must be considered on a case-by-case basis because the symptoms and signs can be varied, and can differ depending on the woman's ethnicity, life stage and even the amount of weight they are carrying. To make things even trickier, the syndrome can also vary over time for an individual.

PCO versus PCOS

Recent reports suggest that 80% of young women (aged 18-22 years old) can have polycystic ovaries (PCO) detected by ultrasound, which decreases in frequency with age [6]. However, only 12-21% of women at reproductive age have the condition PCOS [1]. Thus, healthy women could have polycystic ovaries and experience no other symptoms or only mild symptoms of PCOS and are therefore not diagnosed as having PCOS. Thus, being found to have polycystic ovaries is not sufficient to indicate that you have PCOS. Other tests are required to confirm or dismiss a diagnosis of PCOS.

What tests are used to confirm you have PCOS?

1. The history of a women's menstrual cycle, to determine if her cycle is irregular, infrequent or absent. A period longer than 35 days is often a sign that ovulation (the release of a mature egg from the ovary) has not occurred during the cycle (anovulation). Anovulation can alter the interval, duration or how heavy the bleeding is each cycle. It may also cause either cessation of bleeding or excessive bleeding. Some women (20-50%) can experience regular periods but still not experience ovulation, especially if they have excess androgen levels. Thus, ovulation is often checked by measuring the level of progesterone present in a women's serum (portion of your blood) during the luteal phase of the women's cycle (days 0-10 at the start of a new period).

Keeping track of your menstrual cycle (period)

Track your period by counting the number of days between the first day of your period (when you start to bleed) to the first day of your next period. A menstrual cycle is on average 28 days long, but can range from 21 to 35 days in adults, and 21 to 45 days in young teens. Women with PCOS may have a menstrual cycle that is longer than 35 days or completely absent due to their imbalance of sex hormones and the effect this has on the release of the ovum (egg) during your menstrual cycle.

2. **Hyperandrogenism** (high levels of male sex hormones in your blood) – the biochemical hallmark of PCOS. This often involves examining the physical appearance of a patient and blood tests to assess the level of androgens (male sex hormones) present in the woman's blood. Higher levels of testosterone are commonly found in 80-90% of women experiencing abnormal menstrual cycles [5].

Clinical examination of hyperandrogenism includes looking for the presence of excess hair growth on the face and body, problems with the scalp (dandruff etc.), severe acne on the face but also on other parts of the body like the back and bottom, male pattern balding (top of the head) etc. [8]

The optimal testing method for hyperandrogenism remains controversial. Elevated levels of "free" testosterone (T) account for the majority of PCOS hyperandrogenism cases.

Typically, this is not caused by overproduction of the T but by a decrease in the level of the protein SHBG that normally binds up the "free" T to make it inactive. Insulin and T both have a negative effect on the liver's production of SHBG, creating a negative cycle of allowing more "free" T to circulate around the body.

The most accurate laboratory test used to measure the level of "free" T is a technically challenging and expensive test called equilibrium dialysis. Currently, the best methods commonly available are measurement of "total T" by liquid chromatography-mass spectrometry or RIA methods [1]. In this test, they measure the levels of total T, SHBG and albumin. Then using the known binding affinity (how well it binds to T) of the SHBG and albumin, they can fairly accurately estimate the amount of "free" T that would be present in your blood sample [9].

Because SHBG also binds up estrogen, the reduced levels of SHBG in the blood of PCOS women means that the level of "free" estradiol is often also higher in the blood.

Often the adrenal glands will produce extra precursor steroids that are used to produce androgens (pregnenolone, 17-hydroxypregnenolone, dehydroepiandrosterone (DHEA), androstenedione, 11-deozycortisol and possibly cortisol) [10].

Some PCOS women (25%) also have elevated Dehydroepiandrosterone Sulfate (DHEAS) levels and an even smaller number (10%) have only elevated DHEAS levels with no other abnormal changes to other androgens [5]. High DHEAS levels can cause virilisation in young girls, which causes deepening of the voice, balding, and increased muscle bulk. DHEAS is produced by the adrenal glands and high DHEAS levels may indicate conditions other than PCOS, like adrenal tumours or unusual growth of the adrenal gland (hyperplasia). Because of this, DHEAS levels are not indicative of a specific condition and require other tests to confirm PCOS. DHEAS levels also peak during puberty and decline naturally with age, which would make using this hormone difficult for diagnosing PCOS in young teenage women or post-menopausal women.

Androgens – Why are they so hard to measure?

The medical tests developed to measure the level of testosterone in your blood were generally designed for use in males, where the levels of androgens are naturally a lot higher and easier to assess accurately. The low levels of testosterone and other androgens in women are harder to test accurately in the lower ranges required using current testing methods. To get around this, calculated levels of "free" androgens (not bound to receptors or binding proteins in the blood) are preferred for diagnosis of PCOS. The best time to test this is during a woman's follicular phase of her cycle (start of period until ovulation occurs, ie. 0 -10 day of new period) and in the morning.

Very High Androgen Levels – What else could it be?

Hyperandrogenism is detected in 60-80% of PCOS women. Usually, only small increases outside the normal androgen levels (androstenedione hormone) will be observed. If androgen levels are very high and outside those of the laboratory reference ranges, a secondary cause such as non-classical adrenal hyperplasia may be considered. Adrenal hyperplasia is a rare genetic condition where an enzyme present in the adrenal glands doesn't function properly to convert cholesterol to cortisol, resulting in either excessive or absent production of sex hormones. In some cases this can lead to excess facial hair, virilisation and menstrual irregularity in adolescence along with fertility issues due to anovulation (no release of eggs from ovaries) amongst other symptoms that can present similarly to PCOS. Cushing Syndrome can also cause elevated androgen. It involves a problem with the pituitary gland which signals to the adrenals to produce excess cortisol (stress-related hormone) resulting in high androgen levels. Similarly ovarian and adrenal tumors can result in excess androgen levels.

The pill and getting the correct results in your hormone tests

The oral contraceptive pill makes it difficult to accurately test for the level of androgens (male sex hormones) present in a women's body. This is because the estrogen contained in the pill causes increases in sex hormone binding globulin (SHBG) that reduces the amount of androgen that is available in the body (and for the test). If you were still taking the pill it could appear your levels of bioavailable testosterone, free testosterone and free androgen index is within normal limits. As such, it is recommended that the other methods of contraception be used and the oral contraceptive pill not taken for at least 3 months prior to testing.

3. Ultrasound examination of the ovaries to determine if they are polycystic (having many egg follicles present; PCO). This is usually performed by vaginal ultrasound (see more details of this procedure below), which can look at both the appearance of the ovaries for follicles and also the thickness of the endometrium (the inner layer of cells in the uterus that are normally shed during a woman's period) at the same time.

The ovaries of PCO women often contain 2 to 3 times more maturing egg follicles than that of non-PCO women. However, studies show that these maturing eggs don't die off as quickly as they do in normal ovaries, so it doesn't cause early menopause for women with PCO or PCOS.

The theca cell layer of the ovaries is often thicker (hyperplasia) as is the ovarian cortical layer. Theca cells secrete androgens (like testosterone) in response to insulin and luteinizing hormone (LH). More theca cells or increased activity of the enzyme inside the cells that make androgens results in higher androgen levels in women with PCOS [11].

The inner layer of the uterus, called the endometrium, is often thicker in women with PCOS. This occurs when the uterus is chronically exposed to high levels of estrogen without another sex hormone called progesterone being present (this is often called estrogen dominance). This leads to continued stimulation of the endometrium, which grows more and more layers of cells (hyperplastic; increased number of cells) instead of shedding them regularly during a monthly period.

What is Vaginal Ultrasound?

Vaginal ultrasound examination is reserved for sexually active women only. It is not recommended for adolescents because young girls ovaries often look polycystic because hormonal patterns have not settled into a pattern yet and this may lead to over diagnosis. The method provides a clearer image when compared to abdominal ultrasound, where body fat can prevent clear imaging. It is a safe procedure with only mild discomfort when performed by an experienced ultrasonographer, similar to that experienced during a Pap smear test, but requires longer time to capture all the images required for diagnosis. The procedure is performed in a clinic, where you remove your clothing bottoms and sit in a relaxed position on a reclining chair, using a gown or blanket for modesty. The sterile plastic ultrasound probe (similar in size and shape to a thin curling iron) is then inserted a short distance into your vagina (similar to a tampon) either by you or the ultrasonographer, who then moves the direction of the probe so that they can capture images of the ovaries and uterus.

4. **Gonadotropin levels** – serum luteinizing hormone (LH) is often at normal levels or slightly increased in PCOS women. Follicle-stimulating hormone (FSH) is often lower. This makes the quantities of LH when compared to FSH higher in women with PCOS (often referred to as the LH to FSH ratio).

Gonadotropins are released from the pituitary gland located in your head region and stimulate the release of other hormones from the gonads (ovaries in women).

In order for the tiny follicles inside a woman's ovaries to mature into an ovum (egg) and be release during ovulation, the level of FSH has to rise above a threshold level during the early stage of the menstrual cycle (day 1 -14). This rise in FSH stimulates the maturation of several follicles inside the ovary, which eventually die off and leave one dominant follicle to mature into an ovum (egg). For PCOS women, this rise in FSH is often missing or may be significantly delayed which interferes with ovulation.

For ovulation (release of the mature egg) to occur, a slight drop off and then sudden surge in LH and FSH has to occur (usually around day 14) along with high estrogen levels. Without this coordinated surge, the matured egg can't be released and the endometrium continues to grow under the influence of the high estrogen.

However, LH levels are hard to capture with blood tests due to their quick "pulsatile" release within the body. This makes the measurement of LH and FSH difficult to measure accurately and draw any solid conclusions. As such, the LH: FSH ratio is not usually tested for anymore.

5. **Exclusion Tests** – to check that other conditions are not the reason for similar symptoms. These include a thyroid function test, measurement of prolactin and follicle stimulating hormone (FSH) levels, and measurement of serum 17-hydroxyprogesterone in the follicular phase of the woman's menstrual cycle. These help to rule out thyroid dysfunction, androgen-secreting tumours, Cushing Syndrome, congenital adrenal hyperplasia and hyper-prolactinaemia.

A Positive Diagnosis for PCOS

The Rotterdam criteria (2003)

For a woman to be classified as having the condition of PCOS she must present with two of the following three criteria;

1) Oligo- or Anovulation (periods infrequent or absent),

2) Clinical and/or biochemical signs of hyperandrogenism (high levels of male sex hormones), and

3) Polycystic ovaries (PCO),

Any other causes such as congenital adrenal hyperplasia, androgen-secreting tumours or Cushing's Syndrome that could produce similar symptoms need to be excluded. The three criteria are explained in more detail below along with an explanation of the tests used to confirm them.

Different types of PCOS

For ease of understanding, I've categorised the different forms of PCOS into groups – Type I and II based on the various combinations of criteria you may test positive for in your diagnosis of PCOS. Note - these are not strictly terms used by medical professionals for PCOS.

Type I – **(3/3)** Confirms that you have all three factors present including disrupted menstrual cycles, high levels of androgen (male sex) hormones in your blood (hyperandrogenism) and polycystic ovaries (PCO) diagnosed by ultrasound examination. With all other confounding conditions having been excluded by relevant testing.

Type II – **(2/3)** Confirms you have two of the factors - either A) disrupted menstrual cycle and high levels of androgens but no PCO, B) disrupted menstrual cycle and PCO but not high levels of androgens, or C) high level of androgens and PCO with no apparent disruption to menstrual cycles. Again, with all other confounding conditions having been excluded by relevant testing.

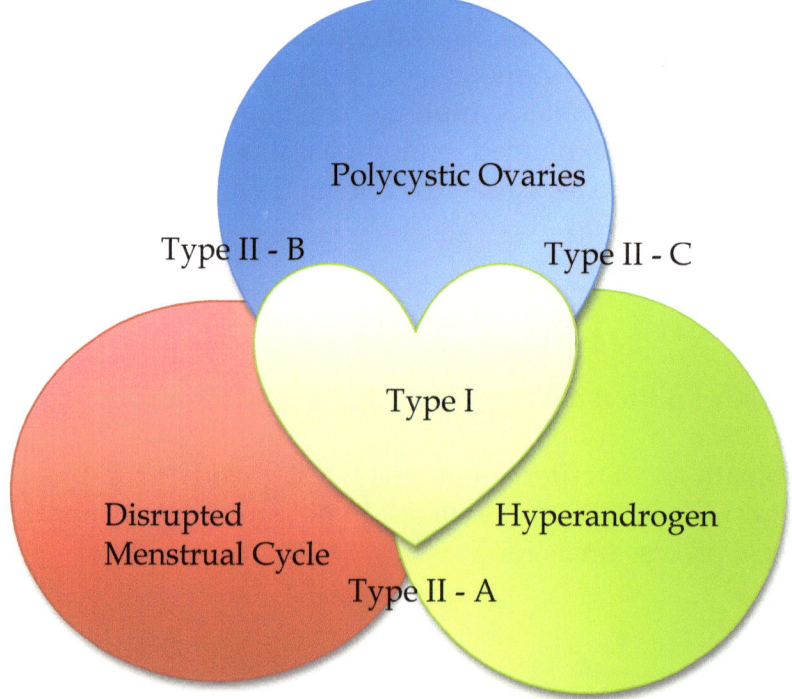

Different Types of PCOS

The new PCOS sisters – Type II B and C

The original National Institute of Health (NIH) and National Institute of Child Health and Human Development (NICHD) criteria only included women with high levels of androgens and disrupted menstrual cycles as candidates for PCOS. Using the new Rotterdam criteria, that includes polycystic ovaries (PCO) as a diagnostic factor, currently means that two new groups of women may be diagnosed with PCOS. They include Type II B - those with PCO and hyperandrogenism without anovulation, and Type II C - those with PCO and chronic anovulation without hyperandrogenism [12].

As such, a distinct group of PCOS women have been identified (Type II B), who have high level androgen hormones (hyperandrogenism) with polycystic ovaries, but experience normal ovulation/menstrual cycles, and thus may be completely unaware that they have PCOS. It appears these women tend to have normal insulin sensitivity and as a result are often leaner than those with "classical" Type I forms of PCOS.

It has been suggested that this ovulatory "slim sister" form of PCOS is a transitional stage between normal and the classical anovulatory form of PCOS. Early lifestyle interventions that help to manage metabolic responses may prevent the full transition from occurring in these women. Despite the apparent regularity of menstruation (monthly periods), these women may not be releasing an egg, making it difficult to get pregnant. They could also be estrogen dominant (low progesterone) making it look like they are producing lots of fertile mucus during the luteal phase of their cycle (day 1-14) and may experience enlarged or sensitive breasts. The high testosterone levels will be producing the classic acne and hair challenges faced by PCOS women. Type II C PCOS ladies are likely to be over sensitive to the effects of androgens rather than producing too much.

Both new forms are likely to carry the same risk of experiencing medical problems associated with PCOS. As such, it is still very important for these women to get the correct testing and diagnosis done, to help them manage their health now and into the future.

Why me? What causes PCOS?

The short answer to this is that we're not sure at the moment. Although the syndrome has been clinically identified since the 1930's, difficulties in accurately assessing whether a woman has high levels of androgens (hyperandrogenism) and other aspects of the condition have made it hard for health professionals to all agree on what are the specific characteristics of PCOS. This has made it hard to research what exactly is causing PCOS. If you don't compare "apples with apples", then the research is not relevant or accurate.

From a small number of research studies that have been done using the Rotterdam criteria for selecting patients in the study, a general belief has emerged that there are both genetic and environmental factors involved in the aetiology (cause) of PCOS. This is explained in more detail in the following section.

It is quite common for a condition to require a genetic predisposition and then an environmental trigger to set the condition in motion. Take coeliac disease as an example, where you may have the gene for coeliac disease but not suffer from the condition until you experience an environmental exposure/trigger like getting a virus or infection in the gut. The environmental trigger then sets off the disease processes (destruction of the gut lining) and you experience symptoms (abdominal discomfort, disrupted bowel movements, poor health etc.).

Likewise in PCOS, environmental triggers such as food, toxins and environmental pollutants may trigger and reveal the genetic tendency to develop PCOS [38].

It isn't clear what directly causes the condition. Medical researchers are currently investigating the syndrome. Research into PCOS hopes to allow better understanding of the condition and aims to find new information and strategies to manage PCOS so you can live a normal, healthy and happy life.

Diagnosis should be viewed as simply the first step in this pathway of better understanding a PCOS woman's body and then a plan can be made on how best to surge forward with your life in the healthiest and most positive ways. In fact, if given the opportunity to participate in any research looking into PCOS, I would encourage you to support medical research to further our knowledge and understanding of the condition.

For interest, the following section will provide a summary of the current understanding of the potential causes of PCOS, but don't get hung up on the lack of definitive answers available at this stage. It is also worth noting that there is not much to be gained from blaming your relatives for your genetic predisposition to PCOS, albeit interesting to understand the potential link. Until the 1980's, PCOS was a rather poorly understood condition. The past 30 years have taught us a great deal, and looking into the future, research that helps us to understand how the disease manifests in our bodies will provide clues and direction for how best to manage or treat the disease and perhaps even prevent the disease from occurring in future generations of women. Research into PCOS has exploded over the past few years and this is very encouraging for the future health of women with PCOS worldwide, so "watch this space" for future updates.

What do we know about the possible causes so far – genetic or environmental?

PCOS is a functional problem that occurs within a woman's endocrine system that causes a disruption to the normal sex hormone levels that are produced in a woman's body. This then leads to the sequence of biological changes and the resulting symptoms that are experienced by women with PCOS (as outlined above), including the appearance of polycystic ovaries. So again, the polycystic ovaries are just one of the symptoms of the condition, not the cause. Currently, it appears that both genetic and environmental factors are important for clinical presentation of PCOS, and that this is also related to the level of obesity, ovarian dysfunction and other factors that influence hormone production or response to hormones in the body.

Genetic factors that could be causing PCOS

Genetics is not the easiest topic to understand, so I'll do my best to give you a brief overview so that you can grasp the basic concepts of how your genetic factors are involved in causing your PCOS condition.

Every part of your body is made up of cells that are joined together in complex ways to form the different parts of your beautiful body to which you have become accustomed since birth. Consider a cell as an extremely small "Lego block" (invisible to the naked eye in fact) that is then used to form different structures.

Within every cell in your body there is a "control centre" called the nucleus that holds the blueprint of the "instruction manual" for the cell. This is where your unique genetic code is to be found. It is all wrapped up in tight spiraling coils called deoxyribonucleic acid (DNA) that are then bundled together in different shaped strands, (that look like wonky strands of tiny rope when viewed under the microscope) that are known as chromosomes.

There are 23 pairs of chromosomes in a human cell (or 46 individual chromosome strands that make up the 23 pairs). Most of the chromosomes (22 pairs) all look the same between males and females except for the 23rd pair, known as the sex chromosomes. If you are male you have both an X and a Y chromosome for the 23rd pair (XY), but if you are female you have two X chromosomes for your 23rd pair (XX).

When "genetic factors" are discussed, what is being referred to is this unique genetic material or "code" contained within the strands of your individual chromosomes. You inherit half of this code from your biological mother (23 chromosomes contained in the egg released from her ovaries) and the other half from your biological father (23 chromosomes contained in the sperm released from his testes), that, when combined at the time of your conception, created the 23 pairs of chromosomes required for humans.

Within these chromosomes, there are thousands of genes, a short sequence of code. These genes have defined and often crucial roles within the cells of your body that make you not only human but also functional (alive!). The combination of different genes sets on the chromosomes is what makes you unique (except in the case of identical twins – where they both have the identical pair of chromosomes).

The genes are read and deciphered by special machinery within the cell that then translates this information into a message (similar to translating a letter written in French into English). This message then controls what the cell produces and enables it to perform its biological role. Many cells can then work together as a tissue (like a team of cells) that go on to form the many larger structures (organs, bones etc.) and essentially these all then function together as a whole system you know as your body.

As such, when researchers say that there are genetic factors identified in a disease such as PCOS, what they mean is that a very tiny part of the genetic material that makes up a particular gene or several genes may have a fault (mistake, missing bits, wrong code etc.) or be different to the general population who don't have the condition. This change in genetics is what then makes that person's cells/organs/body more susceptible to a certain disease condition or may directly cause the condition.

For PCOS, no specific genes have been found to cause the condition in <u>all women</u> with PCOS. Rather, recent studies have shown that changes in several genes can occur in women with PCOS. But frustratingly, the faulty genes within one family can differ to that found in another family of PCOS women. So no single genetic test is available for use as a diagnostic test for all women with PCOS. Conducting more medical research into this may yield answers into the future.

Did I inherit PCOS and, if so, how?

Yes, you can inherit PCOS from your mother or father, but this genetic fault will not necessarily be exactly the same genetic factor found in other PCOS women. However, it can result in the same common symptoms.

PCOS appears to be inherited within families and is believed to be an X-linked dominant disease. This means that the condition is inherited from either parent when they pass on their X-chromosome. As both men (XY) and women (XX) carry an X chromosome in their cells, it means that both a father or mother can pass the condition onto their children, both daughters and sons.

Dominant inheritance means that for females, even though they have two X chromosomes only one of their X-chromosomes has to carry the faulty PCOS gene(s) in order for that woman to present with the disease (eg. X**X** where the bold X represents the PCOS affected X-chromosome).

So daughters (who inherit one X chromosome from their mother and one from their father) of an affected mother (**X**X) and unaffected father (XY) have a 50:50 chance of inheriting the PCOS gene on one of their X-chromosome (**X**X) and being affected like their mother. This means you may have the condition but your sister (XX) may or may not. See the example for "Family One" below.

But if you have a father who is carrying the defective PCOS gene on his X chromosome (**X**Y), then all daughters will inherit PCOS (**X**X) because they have to inherit their fathers affected X chromosome. See the example for "Family Two" below.

No male equivalent of PCOS has been identified. However, a recent study demonstrated that brothers of women with PCOS may also have the metabolic disorders associated with PCOS [13] including imbalance of sugar (glucose) and fat (lipid) levels [14]. Men with metabolic syndrome experience obesity, high blood pressure, high cholesterol, or high blood sugar levels similar to that experienced by PCOS women [15].

Brothers of women with PCOS have also been identified to have increased DHEAS levels, an androgen produced by the adrenal gland, suggesting a similar defect in the over production of androgens similar to their PCOS sisters [16]. Premature male baldness and severe acne is thought to perhaps be one presentation of a PCOS-like condition in men [17].

Example of two family trees showing these inheritance patterns

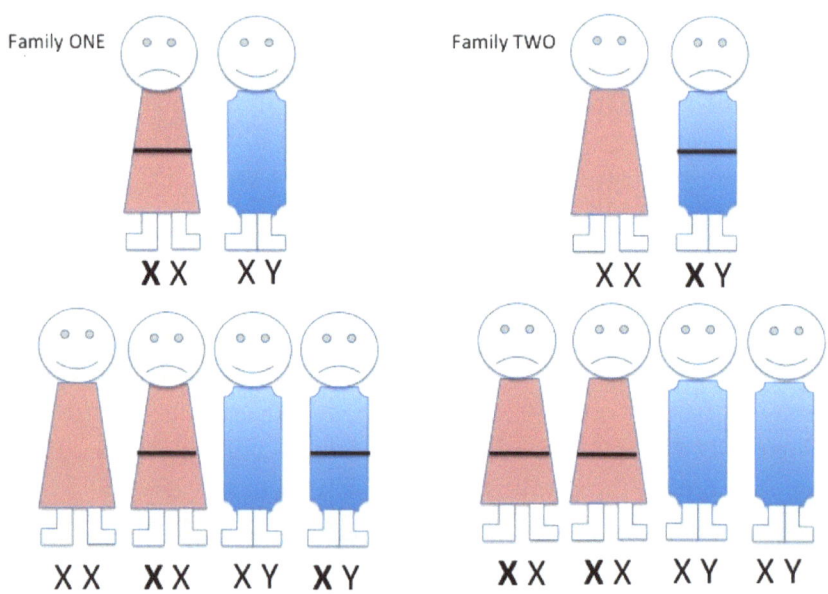

Bold text (X) *is the chromosome carrying the PCOS positive gene, represented in the pictures as a male or female with a sad face and black belt.*

How do researchers identify genetic factors that might be responsible for PCOS?

This next section is a more in depth look at the "how" and "why" of genetic research currently being conducted into the cause of PCOS. Often, to identify if any genetic factors are responsible for a condition, researchers will study the genes present in people with a disease (PCOS for example) and compare them to a group of "control" individuals who are very similar (age/sex/lifestyle etc.) but do not have the disease.

As there are thousands of genes on the 23 pairs of chromosomes contained within human cells, researchers often focus their study on groups of genes that are related to either cellular functions that are not working properly in the disease condition and on the organ(s) that are affected by the disease.

What genes are suspected to play a role in PCOS?

Numerous candidate genes have been proposed to be involved in PCOS [18]. Genetic factors that have been studied by researchers include any relating to sex hormones and their receptors. For example, they have focused on the hormones that stimulate the growth and activity of the sex organs (gonadotropins), the multiple hormones released from the pituitary gland present in the brain that stimulate the function of the ovaries and testes, enzymes important in the making of steroid sex hormones (steroidogenesis), as well as the insulin pathway (regulating sugar/fat metabolism) and its receptors which influence the production of sex hormones. Genes relating to chronic inflammation have also been investigated due to the common presence of low-level chronic inflammation in women with PCOS.

Genes related to hormone induction, production and responses

Hormone Induction: Luteinising hormone (LH) is released in pulses from the pituitary gland in the brain. LH is essential for reproduction as it stimulates the ovaries to make and secrete testosterone, which can then be converted to estrogen by enzymes found in the surrounding granulosa cells. Increased levels of LH are a common finding in women with PCOS. High levels of LH are thought to contribute to poor egg maturation and fertilization, as well as lower pregnancy and higher miscarriage rates [19].

No abnormalities have been found in the gene for LH itself to date, but a mutation that affects the expression of the LH receptor gene has been found [20].

Higher numbers of LH receptors have been detected in some families with PCOS, particularly those with normal LH serum levels but hyperandrogenism at diagnosis [21]. An increased number of receptors on the surface of theca cells make them more sensitive to LH induced steroidogenesis (ie. making more androgen hormones). So the ovary produces more testosterone.

Genes related to the regulation of LH secretion, including Dopamine and Follistatin genes, initially seemed quite promising as genetic target genes, but further studies using larger patient numbers did not find any significant changes to these genes in women with PCOS [22-24].

Hormone production: Increased production and secretion of androgens (like testosterone) is a common occurrence in women with PCOS [25]. There are two enzymes responsible for making these androgen hormones, cytochrome P450 17-hydroxylase (CYP17) and cytochrome P450 side-chain cleavage enzyme (CYP11A). These enzymes are found in the theca cells that make up the outer section of the follicles within the ovary. Research has found that women with "classical" type I PCOS phenotype including hyperandrogenism have increased levels of these enzymes in their follicles [26].

Response to Hormones: The receptors or binding proteins for the sex hormones (mainly testosterone and estrogen) have also been investigated for a possible link to PCOS.
There is a genetic fault in the X-linked androgen receptor (AR; where testosterone binds and causes changes in the target cell) for some PCOS women. This is associated with higher androgen levels but the results remain controversial at this stage [23,27].

The sex hormone binding globulin (SHBG), which is normally present in the blood to "sop up" excess hormones, is often decreased in the serum of women with PCOS. The most likely cause is a genetic fault present in the promoter section (the "start" or "on" section that switches the gene on to produce its product) of the gene for SHBG, which inhibits the production of the SHBG molecule [28]. Interestingly, a recent study has also shown that men with metabolic syndrome (obesity, high blood pressure, high cholesterol, or high blood sugar levels) also have polymorphisms in the SHBG gene[15].

The estrogen receptor (ER) is present in lower numbers in ovarian follicles of women with PCOS compared to healthy women. Studies in mice have shown that mice lacking the estrogen receptor develop PCOS-like disease. Polymorphisms in the estrogen receptor gene are associated with insulin resistance and low FSH levels in women with PCOS. It is considered a genetic modifier of the PCOS phenotype [29].

Insulin or insulin receptor genes in PCOS

Over the last 15 years, studies have confirmed that disrupted insulin pathways play a firm role in the cause of PCOS [9]. *See more details on insulin resistance in the next book of the Health Hunter series: "Management and Treatment of PCOS".* Most women with PCOS, whether lean or obese, have a degree of insulin resistance and compensatory hyper-insulinemia (produce more insulin from their pancreas than is normally required). As such, genes that encode proteins involved in the acquisition or secretion of insulin may play a role.

A recent study involving sisters of women affected with PCOS showed evidence of insulin resistance in all the sisters, suggesting that insulin resistance is a dominant genetic trait among PCOS families, and only some inherit or develop the hyperandrogenism [30] and PCOS syndrome, perhaps through additional environmental or other genetic switches present for the affected sisters. *More details on environmental factors are explained later in this chapter.*

A study in 2002 found a fault in the insulin receptor gene in women with PCOS, but due to small patient numbers this findings were not strong enough to conclude a firm association [31]. A number of studies since have not found any associations with the mutations in the insulin receptor and PCOS. However, this does not rule out functional problems with the insulin pathway as a culprit for insulin resistance in PCOS. Future studies may elucidate this mechanism.

Genes relating to heart disease and chronic inflammation in PCOS

Problems with the cells lining the inside walls of blood vessels and lymphatic vessels (endothelial cells) and increased risk of cardiovascular complications have been associated with PCOS.

Genes like PAI-1 have been found to have a fault in them in a group of Greek women with PCOS [32], and this gene is associated with risk of heart disease and a tendency to experience blood clots in the blood vessels.

Inflammatory signals produced by the fat cells (adipose tissue), including the cytokines TNF□, IL-6 and IL-18 have also been implicated in the disease process of PCOS.
Very interestingly, tumor necrosis factor-alpha (TNF) is secreted by the fat cells and when present in high levels can cause insulin resistance [33]. High levels of TNF are present in the blood of women with PCOS. Genetic faults have been identified in the gene for TNF and also the promoter region of the gene for TNF [34]. In these women, the genetic fault in the TNF gene may be the cause of the insulin resistance, which leads to high levels of insulin present in the blood that then stimulates excess androgen production from the ovaries leading to the symptoms and problems associated with excess testosterone in PCOS women.

The cytokine (chemical messenger) Interleukin-6 (IL-6) is also secreted from fat cells, and promotes the release of C-reactive protein from the liver, which is found to be increased in the blood of obese and women with PCOS [18]. Polymorphisms in the IL-6 gene have been detected in PCOS women from South India [35].

Patients with PCOS also have elevated levels of IL-18 that is linked with cardiovascular disease [36]. However, a study of Chinese women with PCOS showed no correlation the IL-18 gene [37].

It would appear that there are not necessarily genetic faults in the family of pro-inflammatory genes, but rather that there is a preference towards particular alleles of these gene (versions – like blue eyes versus brown eye genes) that could make an individual produce more inflammatory responses [38].

Correcting these genetic anomalies by genetic engineering techniques or blocking the inflammatory signaling pathway with antibodies or small molecule inhibitors may provide future treatments for PCOS women as our medical treatments come of age in the era of enhanced genetic screening and personalised treatment regimes. This is yet another interesting area to watch in the arena of PCOS research.

New genes of interest in PCOS

The human genome, consisting of a map of all the genes present on our 24 sets of chromosomes, was completely mapped out in April 2003. This means that every section of the chromosomes has a unique identification number. Researchers have found that a candidate gene region on chromosome 19p13.2 has been identified in several PCOS families. The region contains the genes for *FNB3* (encoding fibrillin-3), *ELAVL1* (encoding an mRNA-binding protein), and *CCL25* (encoding a thymus expressed chemokine) [39]. More detailed research is currently being conducted on these genes to try to find how they could be linked to PCOS. What we know so far is explained below.

Fibrillin-3 (*FNB3 gene*) is thought to function during the maturation of the follicles that become ovum (eggs) in the ovaries, and a 2010 study found that the factors responsible for generating the fibrillin-3 (transcription factors) were decreased in PCOS women [40]. So perhaps a genetic fault in this part of the genetic code at chromosome 19q is affecting follicle/egg development within the ovaries of women with PCOS. This would disrupt the hormone cycle and result in anovulation, polycystic ovaries and/or hyperandrogenism. Further clinical research is required to confirm these findings.

ELAV-like protein 1 (*ELAVL1 gene*) also known as the human antigen R is a protein that binds the translated genetic message (in the form of RNA) to protect the break down of other genes. Like a bodyguard protecting a client. So it effectively buffers genes from being destroyed by other proteins, meaning that the message for a gene can stay around and keep being made into proteins that serve a function in the cell. If the bodyguard decides to work for evil clients instead of good, then bad things can result.

ELAVL1 has been implicated in cancer and other diseases in the body, where it is overexpressed and hijacked to keep cells alive or functioning in a manner not conducive to normal healthy cells. It is also associated with both pro- and anti-inflammatory responses depending on the type of cell examined.

For women with PCOS, there is also a link between this protein and increased CYP17, the enzyme responsible for androgen production in the theca cells of the ovary. A recent study presented at the 2013 Endocrine Conference by Chen Y, Heneidi S and Azziz R, has shown that ELAVL1 gene is significantly decreased in the fat cells of women with PCOS. What affect this has on inflammatory responses and CYP17 expression remains to be confirmed.

Chemokine (C-C motif) ligand 25 (*CCL25 gene*) – is a small chemical messenger produced by cells (cytokine) that encodes a protein involved in inflammation and regulation of the immune system. It can attract cells of the immune system and other cell types to a location where it is produced (chemoattractant properties) and/or cause cells to mature into different functional types (eg. Monocytes into macrophages) [41]. It has also been found to play a role in the spread of cancer cells, invasion and break-down of tissue structures (by influencing matrix metalloproteinase expression) [42].

Disruptive CCL25 signaling (also known as TECK) has been identified in endometriosis. Misguided CCL25 signals encourage stromal cells from the endometrium to move into regions they don't normally grow [43]. The role of CCL25 in PCOS remains to be determined.

Environmental factors that could be causing PCOS

As mentioned previously, it may be that PCOS is the result of both a genetic element and also an environmental trigger that sets the condition on its course to produce the symptoms you experience. Environmental influences include things that both inside (hormones, metabolism etc.) and outside the body (chemicals, sunlight etc.). The findings of current research into the impact that environmental factors may have in PCOS are detailed below:

Pre-natal and early childhood factors

Some researchers believe that the factors you are exposed to whilst still a growing baby inside your mother's womb can influence your health outcomes as an adult. This may include the levels of sex hormones present in your mother's body, her diet, your gestational growth and your weight at birth. These are explained in more detail below and include both clinical research findings and also those artificially produced in experimental animal models of PCOS.

Levels of Testosterone: Exposure to high levels of the sex hormone testosterone whilst still in the womb may lead to PCOS in female children. Despite some animal models which show a link between high testosterone exposure and PCOS like symptoms in young female babies [44-48], it is unlikely that these slightly elevated levels of testosterone present in pregnant PCOS women would reach the child *in utero*. This is because the placenta was found to produce enzymes (placental aromatase) that provide a barrier against the mother's androgens [49,50]. This study also examined the level of testosterone present in the blood of pregnant PCOS mothers in the middle and the end of their pregnancy, and in the cord blood from the baby, but showed no relationship with the later development of PCOS in the children.

Outcome of Birth Weight: An interesting hypothesis called the "Barker hypothesis" or "the fetal origins hypothesis" suggests that low birth weight (evidence of restricted growth in the womb) causes insulin resistance, cardiovascular disease and other features of insulin resistance syndrome [51-53]. In this case, insulin resistance is considered the result of compensation mechanisms because of decreased nutrient supply to the baby.

However, other studies have shown that babies born with large birth weights such as those born to mothers with gestational diabetes, can also have poor metabolic outcomes as adults [54]. Two studies have been performed to examine this idea. One study has found an association between mothers with PCOS having babies that were large for gestational age compared to non-PCOS women [50]. However, larger studies have since not shown any link between birth weight and development of PCOS in later life [55].

Studies that examined children of PCOS women before they reached puberty, suggest that PCOS has effects on metabolic functions long before the reproductive effects become apparent. These include higher testosterone levels and anti-Mullerian hormone levels (a marker of ovarian follicle numbers), hyper-insulinemia, higher leptin levels and lower adiponectin levels in daughters prior to reaching puberty. Similarly, the sons of women with PCOS tended to have higher levels of testosterone and were heavier during their infancy [56].

Fat metabolism and obesity

There are not too many women who can say that they haven't battled with their weight at some stage in their life. But for women with PCOS the battle can be super frustrating when the normal methods for managing your weight don't seem to work for them. This can lead to a situation where fat builds up over the years and your body-mass-index (BMI; a simple index of weight-to-height ratio) continues to slide up and up.

When a woman's BMI peaks over 25, she is regarded as overweight and if it reaches over 30 then she is classified as obese. For every woman, regardless of her PCOS status, being overweight or obese puts tremendous stress on her body, leading to a greater risk of death from cardiovascular disease, diabetes and cancers.

So, why should you care about your weight? It's not about how you look. Being overweight or obese makes your PCOS symptoms worse, including elevating your already high androgen levels, balding, excess hair growth, infertility and other complications arising during pregnancy [57,58]. It is also now understood that obesity is associated with low-grade chronic inflammation[59]. Evidence for this comes from studies that have shown the biological markers of inflammation (TNF, C-reactive protein, and interleukins etc.) are elevated in women with PCOS but the results of these studies are still quite controversial.

Inflammation is an immune response designed to help the body defend against injury or disease. Chronic inflammation, on the other hand, is a disease, turning a good situation into a bad one. Chronic inflammation contributes substantially to disease such as cancer and cardiovascular disease. What is clear is that obesity escalates your already heightened risk of certain health complications, including cardiovascular disease, diabetes and impaired glucose tolerance [60].

Understanding how the body stores and releases fat to balance the body's need for energy is very important for women with PCOS. The reality is you probably will have to work harder or smarter (or both) than the average woman to keep your weight in check. The hope is that this information helps you to understand how PCOS may be causing the challenges you are facing and then allow you to be smarter about your food and lifestyle choices so that you start to see results, can set realistic weight loss goals, and work towards a healthier and happier you.

More details on weight management strategies are included in part two of this *Health Hunter Books* series "Enlightened Guide to PCOS: Management and Treatment Options for PCOS".

It is also very important to note that, like all other aspects of PCOS, not all women with PCOS will have issues with their weight. What this means is that it is highly unlikely that obesity is the cause of PCOS; rather, it may be the consequence of PCOS-related changes that lead to a dysfunctional weight management system for your body.

Although 50 to 80% of PCOS women struggle with weight issues, obesity is not a problem for every individual with PCOS, particularly the newly diagnosed Type II B and C "slim sisters". The percentage of obese women with PCOS varies from country to country, suggesting that genetic as well as environmental factors such as lifestyle and diet may contribute significantly to obesity in women with PCOS [9]. As the rate of obesity is rising in the population worldwide, there is no evident increase in the number of women being diagnosed with PCOS [61]. There are also many lean women affected by PCOS. Innovative research into this topic has revealed some exciting new findings that help us to understand how PCOS can alter the balance of fat use versus storage in our bodies.

Current findings suggest that there may be biological changes associated with obesity in women with PCOS. Firstly, the cells that store fat (adipocytes) examined from women with PCOS (both lean and obese women) were found to be physically larger in size. Secondly, there are problems with how fat moves in and out of the cells [62]. Lastly, women with PCOS may also have lower levels of the insulin sensitizing chemokine, called adiponectin, compared to reproductively normal women. Both enlarged fat cells and low serum adiponectin levels are strongly associated with insulin resistance[63]. This provides strong evidence for a mechanism by which PCOS women develop insulin resistance leading to chronic weight gain and eventually obesity [64].

Another potential problem for PCOS women with regard to energy balance, hormone balance and weight management is the development of leptin resistance. Leptin is a cytokine (chemical messenger for cells) from the tumor necrosis factor (TNF) family. It is released from fat cells (adipocytes) in a pulsatile pattern and controls appetite by telling the brain that it has sufficient energy stores (ie. stop eating now) and thermogenesis (body warmth).

The levels of leptin directly relate to the quantity of fat stored in the body. Leptin induces the break down of fat cells to release the fat stores (a process known as lipolysis). It is released in response to insulin signals that come from the pancreas during states of low energy/glucose levels (in between meals, during exercise etc.) to ensure the constant availability of energy for the vital organs of the body like the brain. Leptin also regulates food intake by activating the leptin receptors present on the hypothalamus section of the brain and causing a reduction in food intake urges.

High levels of leptin are thought to contribute to a state of leptin resistance, where the brain does not respond to the leptin signals appropriately, so the body produces higher levels to compensate. That makes it harder for a person to stop eating, even after their body has had enough.

Leptin is also involved in reproductive functions of the body. Leptin receptors are also found on granulosa and theca cells within the follicles of the ovary. Chronic high-level exposure to leptin causes the ovaries to stop producing steroid sex hormones and subsequently blocks ovulation.

For women with PCOS, using the diabetic treatment drug metformin has resulted in successful weight loss, lower BMI, reduction in fasting blood glucose levels and insulin, reduced testosterone and leptin with an increased progesterone production, which results in increased ovulation and pregnancy rates.

Similar results are found in lean PCOS women, suggesting that excess leptin or hypersensitivity to leptin may be caused by factors other than obesity [65], genetic changes in the leptin receptors or environmental toxins that mimic the effects of leptin.

Nutritional deficiency

Vitamin D is a fat-soluble precursor for a steroid hormone called calcitriol. Vitamin D is naturally acquired from exposure to UV radiation from the sun and is important for absorption of calcium and phosphate to provide strong and healthy bones and muscles. Several recent studies have looked at a link between vitamin D levels in blood and PCOS, in particular insulin resistance in PCOS women.

Studies suggest that lower levels of vitamin D correlate with metabolic disturbances including insulin resistance in PCOS [66]. However, a recent study has shown no benefit for insulin resistance by supplementation with 50,000IU of vitamin D3 for 2 months for PCOS women with insulin resistance [67].

It has been suggested that abnormalities in ovarian follicular development may be caused by an imbalance in calcium. One study found that women with irregular periods that were treated with vitamin D and calcium supplements experienced a more normal cycle after 2 months of treatment, and some even became pregnant during the study [68].

Overweight women with PCOS, also saw improved blood pressure and lower androgen profiles after daily supplementation with vitamin D and calcium for 3 months, but had no effect on insulin resistance or glucose homeostasis [69].

However, a recent systematic review of the topic found it hard to draw any strong conclusions, and suggested that more appropriate well-designed clinical trials are required to confirm any firm links [70].

Medication-induced PCOS

Medications such as anticonvulsant drugs used for the treatment of epilepsy can cause endocrine disorders including the development of PCOS [71]. Please consult your general practitioner or specialist before considering changes to your current medication.

Living to your full potential with PCOS

Congratulations! You've just taken a huge step in the path to your future health and happiness as a woman who not only lives with PCOS but also thrives and strives to live to her full potential every day. A diagnosis of PCOS should not be a devastating event. In fact, it should be an enlightening moment that gives you the opportunity to understand what is occurring in your body and why it produces the effects it does. I'm sure there was lots of "Ah-haaa! That's why..." moments for you when you read through the list of possible symptoms. More importantly, being diagnosed with PCOS should also be the moment you can start taking steps to get your health back on track and enable you to live to your full potential.

PCOS is an incredibly common condition, and although it is not fully understood just yet, the information we have gained through research and medical studies is already very empowering. It means we can now make changes based on an understanding of how this can restore balance to the body that results in positive outcomes in your health. Being aware not only of what physical changes are occurring in your body but also what mental effects these may be having on you can help you to take stock, adjust your mindset to allow you to come to grips with the diagnosis, and then move forward to make a personal plan to improve your health and happiness.

Importantly, since the diagnosis criteria for PCOS is now more clearly defined and universally applied, new knowledge (through research) has identified several related health concerns for women with PCOS, including heart disease, cancers and diabetes. So correct diagnosis and on going monitoring is more important than ever.

You probably discovered the *Health Hunter Books* series because you were searching for answers and support. There are also several other organisations within Australia that provide excellent resources and support for women with Polycystic Ovarian Syndrome (PCOS). These include (but are not limited to) to Jean Hailes women's health organisation http://www.jeanhailes.org.au, which provides information and support for numerous women's health issues, and the Polycystic Ovarian Syndrome Association of Australia (POSAA), established in 1988 as a "self help" information and support group for Australian women with PCOS http://www.posaa.asn.au.

There is also a growing tribe of social media sites, including http://www.pcosdiva.com, that provide excellent information and exciting new research findings. Whether I recommend a site or not, I would like to let you know that I am in no way affiliated with these companies or individuals. I will not be making money if you visit these sites, and they have not paid for advertising in this e-book. This e-book is for you, and there are no strings attached.

Concluding remarks

What is of utmost importance now is for you to obtain a thorough personal diagnosis of PCOS so you can clearly understand the specific ways your body is operating out of balance as a result of PCOS. You can then use various lifestyle management strategies and/or medical interventions devised by your professional health team (doctors, nutritionists, psychologists etc.) to target these specific changes and restore balance and ultimately let you live your life to the max.

I know this new knowledge will help you to become Powerfully Capable of Obtaining Success (my preferred PCOS title) in anything you set your mind to, rather than focusing on the potentially worrisome and negative aspects of being diagnosed with PCOS.

You are not alone. You are part of a very special group of women and now, with this new knowledge, you can obtain or maintain your beautiful strong balanced mind and body, and more importantly stay healthy and happy.

Thank you for reading. If you found this eBook useful we'd love you to share it with other PCOS women and if you like, leave a comment on our webpage or social media sites. Even better, you could leave a review Amazon or on your eBook retailer site.

Other e-books in the Health Hunter Books series

Enlightening Guide to PCOS: Treatment and Management Strategies for Polycystic Ovarian Syndrome. *Author: Dr. Linda J Howland (PhD) – COMING SOON***

Enlightening Guide to PCOS: Fertility and Aging for women with Polycystic Ovarian Syndrome. *Author: Dr. Linda J Howland (PhD) – COMING SOON***

** Join the mailing list at your favourite book retailer to keep informed on publication release dates and why not leave a review of this book at the same time.

Join the conversation

References

1. Teede, H. J. *et al.* Assessment and management of polycystic ovary syndrome: summary of an evidence-based guideline. *Med. J. Aust.* 195, S65–112 (2011).

2. March, W. A. *et al.* The prevalence of polycystic ovary syndrome in a community sample assessed under contrasting diagnostic criteria. *Hum. Reprod.* 25, 544–551 (2010).

3. Legro, R. S. & Strauss, J. F. Molecular progress in infertility: polycystic ovary syndrome. *Fertil. Steril.* 78, 569–576 (2002).

4. Baghdadi, L. R. *et al.* Impact of obesity on reproductive outcomes after ovarian ablative therapy in PCOS: a collaborative meta-analysis. *Reprod. Biomed. Online* 25, 227–241 (2012).

5. Azziz, R. *et al.* The Androgen Excess and PCOS Society criteria for the polycystic ovary syndrome: the complete task force report. *Fertil. Steril.* 91, 456–488 (2009).

6. Pasquali, R. *et al.* PCOS Forum: research in polycystic ovary syndrome today and tomorrow. *Clin. Endocrinol. (Oxf)* 74, 424–433 (2011).

7. Meenakumari, K. J., Agarwal, S., Krishna, A. & Pandey, L. K. Effects of metformin treatment on luteal phase progesterone concentration in polycystic ovary syndrome. *Braz. J. Med. Biol. Res.* 37, 1637–1644 (2004).

8. DeVane, G. W., Czekala, N. M., Judd, H. L. & Yen, S. S. Circulating gonadotropins, estrogens, and androgens in polycystic ovarian disease. *Am. J. Obstet. Gynecol.* 121, 496–500 (1975).

9. Diamanti-Kandarakis, E. & Dunaif, A. Insulin resistance and the polycystic ovary syndrome revisited: an update on mechanisms and implications. *Endocr. Rev.* 33, 981–1030 (2012).

10. Yildiz, B. O. & Azziz, R. The adrenal and polycystic ovary syndrome. *Rev Endocr Metab Disord* 8, 331–342 (2007).

11. Webber, L. J. *et al.* Prolonged survival in culture of preantral follicles from polycystic ovaries. *J. Clin. Endocrinol. Metab.* 92, 1975–1978 (2007).

12. Azziz, R. *et al.* Positions statement: criteria for defining polycystic ovary syndrome as a predominantly hyperandrogenic syndrome: an Androgen Excess Society guideline. *J. Clin. Endocrinol. Metab.* 91, 4237–4245 (2006).

13. Urbanek, M., Sam, S., Legro, R. S. & Dunaif, A. Identification of a polycystic ovary syndrome susceptibility variant in fibrillin-3 and association with a metabolic phenotype. *J. Clin. Endocrinol. Metab.* 92, 4191–4198 (2007).

14. Sam, S., Sung, Y.-A., Legro, R. S. & Dunaif, A. Evidence for pancreatic beta-cell dysfunction in brothers of women with polycystic ovary syndrome. *Metab. Clin. Exp.* 57, 84–89 (2008).

15. Xita, N. *et al.* The (TAAAA)n polymorphism of the SHBG gene in men with the metabolic syndrome. *Exp. Clin. Endocrinol. Diabetes* 119, 126–128 (2011).

16. Legro, R. S. *et al.* Elevated dehydroepiandrosterone sulfate levels as the reproductive phenotype in the brothers of women with polycystic ovary syndrome. *J. Clin. Endocrinol. Metab.* 87, 2134–2138 (2002).

17. Govind, A., Obhrai, M. S. & Clayton, R. N. Polycystic ovaries are inherited as an autosomal dominant trait: analysis of 29 polycystic ovary syndrome and 10 control families. *J. Clin. Endocrinol. Metab.* 84, 38–43 (1999).

18. Kosova, G. & Urbanek, M. Genetics of the polycystic ovary syndrome. *Mol. Cell. Endocrinol.* 373, 29–38 (2013).

19. Rotterdam ESHRE/ASRM-Sponsored PCOS Consensus Workshop Group. Revised 2003 consensus on diagnostic criteria and long-term health risks related to polycystic ovary syndrome. *Fertil. Steril.* 81, 19–25 (2004).

20. Mutharasan, P. *et al.* Evidence for chromosome 2p16.3 polycystic ovary syndrome susceptibility locus in affected women of European ancestry. *J. Clin. Endocrinol. Metab.* 98, E185–90 (2013).

21. Comim, F. V., Teerds, K., Hardy, K. & Franks, S. Increased protein expression of LHCG receptor and 17□-hydroxylase/17-20-lyase in human polycystic ovaries. *library.newcastle.edu.au*

22. Kahsar-Miller, M., Boots, L. R. & Azziz, R. Dopamine D3 receptor polymorphism is not associated with the polycystic ovary syndrome. *Fertil. Steril.* 71, 436–438 (1999).

23. Urbanek, M. *et al.* Allelic variants of the follistatin gene in polycystic ovary syndrome. *J. Clin. Endocrinol. Metab.* 85, 4455–4461 (2000).

24. Urbanek, M. *et al.* Variation in resistin gene promoter not associated with polycystic ovary syndrome. *Diabetes* 52, 214–217 (2003).

25. Laven, J. S. E., Imani, B., Eijkemans, M. J. C. & Fauser, B. C. J. M. New approach to polycystic ovary syndrome and other forms of anovulatory infertility. *Obstet Gynecol Surv* 57, 755–767 (2002).

26. Wickenheisser, J. K. *et al.* Differential activity of the cytochrome P450 17alpha-hydroxylase and steroidogenic acute regulatory protein gene promoters in normal and polycystic ovary syndrome theca cells. *J. Clin. Endocrinol. Metab.* 85, 2304–2311 (2000).

27. Mifsud, A., Ramirez, S. & Yong, E. L. Androgen receptor gene CAG trinucleotide repeats in anovulatory infertility and polycystic ovaries. *J. Clin. Endocrinol. Metab.* 85, 3484–3488 (2000).

28. Xita, N., Tsatsoulis, A., Chatzikyriakidou, A. & Georgiou, I. Association of the (TAAAA)n repeat polymorphism in the sex hormone-binding globulin (SHBG) gene with polycystic ovary syndrome and relation to SHBG serum levels. *J. Clin. Endocrinol. Metab.* 88, 5976–5980 (2003).

29. Nectaria, X., Leandros, L., Ioannis, G. & Agathocles, T. The importance of ER□ and ER□ gene polymorphisms in PCOS. *Gynecol. Endocrinol.* 28, 505–508 (2012).

30. Diamanti-Kandarakis, E. & Alexandraki, K. Presence of metabolic risk factors in non-obese PCOS sisters: evidence of heritability of insulin resistance. *Journal of Endocrinol. Invest.* (2004).

31. Siegel, S. *et al.* A C/T single nucleotide polymorphism at the tyrosine kinase domain of the insulin receptor gene is associated with polycystic ovary syndrome. *Fertil. Steril.* 78, 1240–1243 (2002).

32. Diamanti-Kandarakis, E. & Palioniko, G. The prevalence of 4G5G polymorphism of plasminogen activator inhibitor-1 (PAI-1) gene in polycystic ovarian syndrome and its association with plasma PAI-1 levels. *European Journal of Endocrinology* (2004).

33. Hotamisligil, G. S. The role of TNFalpha and TNF receptors in obesity and insulin resistance. *J. Intern. Med.* 245, 621–625 (1999).

34. Yun, J.-H., Choi, J.-W., Lee, K.-J., Shin, J.-S. & Baek, K.-H. The promoter -1031(T/C) polymorphism in tumor necrosis factor-alpha associated with polycystic ovary syndrome. *Reprod. Biol. Endocrinol.* 9, 131 (2011).

35. Tumu, V. R. *et al.* An interleukin-6 gene promoter polymorphism is associated with polycystic ovary syndrome in South Indian women. *J. Assist. Reprod. Genet.* (2013). doi:10.1007/s10815-013-0111-1

36. Kaya, C., Pabuccu, R., Berker, B. & Satiroglu, H. Plasma interleukin-18 levels are increased in the polycystic ovary syndrome: relationship of carotid intima-media wall thickness and cardiovascular risk factors. *Fertil. Steril.* 93, 1200–1207 (2010).

37. Yang, Y., Qiao, J. & Li, M. Association of polymorphisms of interleukin-18 gene promoter region with polycystic ovary syndrome in chinese population. *Reprod. Biol. Endocrinol.* (2010).

38. Diamanti-Kandarakis, E. *et al.* Polycystic ovary syndrome: the influence of environmental and genetic factors. *Hormones (Athens)* 5, 17–34 (2006).

39. Urbanek, M. *et al.* Candidate gene region for polycystic ovary syndrome on chromosome 19p13.2. *J. Clin. Endocrinol. Metab.* 90, 6623–6629 (2005).

40. Jordan, C. D., Bohling, S. D., Charbonneau, N. L. & Sakai, L. Y. Fibrillins in Adult Human Ovary and Polycystic Ovary Syndrome: Is Fibrillin-3 Affected in PCOS? *Journal of Histochemistry & Cytochemistry* 58, 903–915 (2010).

41. Schmutz, C. *et al.* Monocytes/macrophages express chemokine receptor CCR9 in rheumatoid arthritis and CCL25 stimulates their differentiation. *Arthritis Res. Ther.* 12, R161 (2010).

42. Johnson-Holiday, C. *et al.* CCL25 mediates migration, invasion and matrix metalloproteinase expression by breast cancer cells in a CCR9-dependent fashion. *Int. J. Oncol.* 38, 1279–1285 (2011).

43. Wang, Y. *et al.* Abnormal regulation of chemokine TECK and its receptor CCR9 in the endometriotic milieu is involved in pathogenesis of endometriosis by way of enhancing invasiveness of endometrial stromal cells. *Cell. Mol. Immunol.* 7, 51–60 (2010).

44. Dumesic, D. A., Abbott, D. H. & Padmanabhan, V. Polycystic ovary syndrome and its developmental origins. *Rev Endocr Metab Disord* 8, 127–141 (2007).

45. Abbott, D. H., Tarantal, A. F. & Dumesic, D. A. Fetal, infant, adolescent and adult phenotypes of polycystic ovary syndrome in prenatally androgenized female rhesus monkeys. *Am. J. Primatol.* 71, 776–784 (2009).

46. Abbott, D. H., Barnett, D. K., Bruns, C. M. & Dumesic, D. A. Androgen excess fetal programming of female reproduction: a developmental aetiology for polycystic ovary syndrome? *Hum. Reprod. Update* 11, 357–374 (2005).

47. Demissie, M. *et al.* Transient prenatal androgen exposure produces metabolic syndrome in adult female rats. *Am. J. Physiol. Endocrinol. Metab.* 295, E262–8 (2008).

48. Foecking, E. M., Szabo, M., Schwartz, N. B. & Levine, J. E. Neuroendocrine consequences of prenatal androgen exposure in the female rat: absence of luteinizing hormone surges, suppression of progesterone receptor gene expression, and acceleration of the gonadotropin-releasing hormone pulse generator. *Biol. Reprod.* 72, 1475–1483 (2005).

49. Nagamani, M., McDonough, P. G., Ellegood, J. O. & Mahesh, V. B. Maternal and amniotic fluid steroids throughout human pregnancy. *Am. J. Obstet. Gynecol.* 134, 674–680 (1979).

50. Anderson, H. *et al.* Infants of women with polycystic ovary syndrome have lower cord blood androstenedione and estradiol levels. *J. Clin. Endocrinol. Metab.* 95, 2180–2186 (2010).

51. Breier, B. H., Vickers, M. H., Ikenasio, B. A., Chan, K. Y. & Wong, W. P. Fetal programming of appetite and obesity. *Mol. Cell. Endocrinol.* 185, 73–79 (2001).

52. Godfrey, K. M. Maternal regulation of fetal development and health in adult life. *Eur. J. Obstet. Gynecol. Reprod. Biol.* 78, 141–150 (1998).

53. Godfrey, K. M. & Barker, D. J. Fetal programming and adult health. *Public Health Nutr* 4, 611–624 (2001).

54. Silverman, B. L., Rizzo, T. A., Cho, N. H. & Metzger, B. E. Long-term effects of the intrauterine environment. The Northwestern University Diabetes in Pregnancy Center. *Diabetes Care* 21 Suppl 2, B142–9 (1998).

55. Hickey, M. *et al.* The relationship between maternal and umbilical cord androgen levels and polycystic ovary syndrome in adolescence: a prospective cohort study. *J. Clin. Endocrinol. Metab.* 94, 3714–3720 (2009).

56. Kent, S. C. *et al.* Hyperandrogenism and hyperinsulinism in children of women with polycystic ovary syndrome: a controlled study. *J. Clin. Endocrinol. Metab.* 93, 1662–1669 (2008).

57. Balen, A. H., Conway, G. S., Kaltsas, G. & Techatraisak, K. Andrology: Polycystic ovary syndrome: the spectrum of the disorder in 1741 patients. *Human ...* (1995).

58. Kiddy, D. S. *et al.* Differences in clinical and endocrine features between obese and non-obese subjects with polycystic ovary syndrome: an analysis of 263 consecutive cases. *Clin. Endocrinol. (Oxf)* 32, 213–220 (1990).

59. Rashad, N. M., El-Shal, A. S. & Abdelaziz, A. M. Association between inflammatory biomarker serum procalcitonin and obesity in women with polycystic ovary syndrome. *J. Reprod. Immunol.* 97, 232–239 (2013).

60. Teede, H., Deeks, A. & Moran, L. Polycystic ovary syndrome: a complex condition with psychological, reproductive and metabolic manifestations that impacts on health across the lifespan. *BMC Med* 8, 41 (2010).

61. Yildiz, B. O., Knochenhauer, E. S. & Azziz, R. Impact of obesity on the risk for polycystic ovary syndrome. *J. Clin. Endocrinol. Metab.* 93, 162–168 (2008).

62. Faulds, G., Rydén, M., Ek, I., Wahrenberg, H. & Arner, P. Mechanisms behind lipolytic catecholamine resistance of subcutaneous fat cells in the polycystic ovarian syndrome. *J. Clin. Endocrinol. Metab.* 88, 2269–2273 (2003).

63. Mannerås-Holm, L. *et al.* Adipose tissue has aberrant morphology and function in PCOS: enlarged adipocytes and low serum adiponectin, but not circulating sex steroids, are strongly associated with insulin resistance. *J. Clin. Endocrinol. Metab.* 96, E304–11 (2011).

64. Berg, A. H., Combs, T. P., Du, X., Brownlee, M. & Scherer, P. E. The adipocyte-secreted protein Acrp30 enhances hepatic insulin action. *Nat. Med.* 7, 947–953 (2001).

65. Upadhyaya, P., Rehan, H. S. & Seth, V. Serum leptin changes with metformin treatment in polycystic ovarian syndrome: correlation with ovulation, insulin and testosterone levels. *EXCLI J* (2011).

66. Mahmoudi, T. Genetic variation in the vitamin D receptor and polycystic ovary syndrome risk. *Fertil. Steril.* 92, 1381–1383 (2009).

67. Ardabili, H. R., Gargari, B. P. & Farzadi, L. Vitamin D supplementation has no effect on insulin resistance assessment in women with polycystic ovary syndrome and vitamin D deficiency. *Nutr Res* 32, 195–201 (2012).

68. Thys-Jacobs, S., Donovan, D., Papadopoulos, A., Sarrel, P. & Bilezikian, J. P. Vitamin D and calcium dysregulation in the polycystic ovarian syndrome. *Steroids* 64, 430–435 (1999).

69. Pal, L. *et al.* Therapeutic implications of vitamin D and calcium in overweight women with polycystic ovary syndrome. *Gynecol. Endocrinol.* 28, 965–968 (2012).

70. Krul-Poel, Y. H. *et al.* The role of vitamin D in metabolic disturbances in polycystic ovary syndrome (PCOS): a systematic review. *Eur. J. Endocrinol.* (2013). doi:10.1530/EJE-13-0617

71. Ayyagari, M., Chitela, S. R. & Kolachana, V. Obesity, polycystic ovarian syndrome and thyroid dysfunction in women with epilepsy. *Ann Indian Acad Neurol* 15, 101–105 (2012).

www.ingramcontent.com/pod-product-compliance
Lightning Source LLC
Chambersburg PA
CBHW050816290526
45792CB00001B/136